EVERYTHING ABOUT

LOW GLYCEMIC

DIET

Complete Nutritional Cookbook, Foods, Meal Plan, Recipes To Weight Loss, Blood Sugar And Insulin Control, Immune Support, Boost Energy, And Enhanced Mood

DR. ALVIN BRANTLEY

Disclaimer

The information provided in this book is intended for general informational purposes only. It is not a substitute for professional medical advice, diagnosis, or treatment.

You should not use the information in this book for diagnosing or treating a health problem or disease by self decision. Always seek the advice of your physician or other qualified health provider with any questions you may have regarding a medical condition.

The author and publisher of this book make no representations or warranties with respect to the accuracy, applicability, fitness, or completeness of the contents of this book. The information contained in this book is based on the author's research and experience, and it is shared with the understanding that the author is not engaged in rendering medical, health, or any other kind of professional advice for you by this book.

The author does not endorse or promote any specific products, brands, or companies related to the contents provided in this book.

Any mention of products or services in this book is for informational purposes only and does not constitute an endorsement.

The author has not entered into any affiliate marketing agreements and has not signed any endorsement deals with individuals, organizations, or companies.

Readers are encouraged to consult with their healthcare providers before making any dietary or lifestyle chaSnges based on the information provided in this book. The author and publisher disclaim any liability for the decisions made by readers based on the information in this book.

Contents

Introduction

Keeping blood sugar levels steady is critical for general health and well-being. Blood sugar fluctuations can cause several health problems, such as diabetes, obesity, and cardiovascular disorders. The Low Glycemic Load Diet, which emphasizes eating foods that have little effect on blood sugar levels, is one useful strategy for controlling blood sugar levels. Rather than focusing solely on the glycemic index, this dietary approach highlights the kind of carbs and how they affect the glycemic load.

An Overview of the Diet with Low Glycemic Load

The goal of the Low Glycemic Load Diet is to assist people in controlling their blood sugar levels by selecting meals that have a lower glycemic load. The glycemic load takes into account both the amount and quality of carbohydrates in a particular meal, in contrast to the glycemic index, which gauges how quickly they elevate blood sugar. People can lower their chance of developing insulin resistance and maintain stable blood sugar levels by adopting this strategy into their dietary habits.

The Value of Consistent Blood Sugar Levels

Blood sugar levels that are stable are essential for general health and are important for both controlling and avoiding several medical disorders. A blood sugar rise and collapse can include heightened appetite, agitation, exhaustion, and trouble focusing. Moreover, type 2 diabetes, insulin resistance, and inflammation are linked to persistently high blood sugar levels. By encouraging a sustainable and balanced approach to carbohydrate consumption, the Low Glycemic Load Diet helps to manage weight, boost energy levels, and maintain long-term metabolic health.

Important Guidelines for the Low-Glycemic Load Diet

The Low Glycemic Load Diet places a strong emphasis on several fundamental ideas to assist people in choosing better foods and preserving stable blood sugar levels. These guidelines include eating meals high in fiber, choosing complex carbs over simple sweets, and watching portion sizes. Through knowledge of the glycemic load of various foods and wise choice-making, people can design a balanced, fulfilling diet that promotes steady blood sugar levels all day long.

Selecting Foods with Low Glycemic Load

People who follow the Low-Glycemic Load Diet should concentrate on including a range of low-glycemic-load items in their meals. Lean proteins, fruits, vegetables, whole grains, and legumes are a few of these. These nutrient-dense choices give you long-lasting energy without sharp blood sugar spikes and crashes. Furthermore, adding good fats can improve satiety even more and help keep the diet balanced overall.

Organizing Meals and Recipes

One of the main components of the Low Glycemic Load Diet is efficient meal planning. People can maintain stable blood sugar levels by preparing well-balanced meals that include a variety of low-glycemic carbohydrates, proteins, and fats. While guaranteeing that nutritional objectives are fulfilled, meal planning ahead of time and experimenting with low-glycemic-load recipes can bring interest and variation to the diet. Additionally, this method makes it easier to regulate ingredient selection and portion amounts.

Possible Advantages of a Low-Glycemic Load Diet

Beyond just balancing blood sugar, the Low Glycemic Load Diet may have several other positive health effects. Improved insulin sensitivity, better weight control, and a lower chance of type 2 diabetes are a few possible benefits.

Furthermore, the diet's emphasis on whole, nutrient-dense foods improves general nutrition, promoting the best possible health and well-being.

Obstacles and Things to Think About

Despite the Low Glycemic Load Diet's demonstrated advantages, it's important to be aware of any potential drawbacks and concerns.

These could include the requirement for regular meal planning, possible dietary restrictions, and individual differences in glycemic reactivity.

People who are aware of these factors will be able to successfully follow the diet and modify it as necessary to fit their tastes and way of life.

The Low Glycemic Load Diet provides a workable and long-term strategy for encouraging stable blood sugar levels. People can experience increased energy, better weight control, and long-term metabolic health by choosing carefully what they eat, including a range of nutrient-dense foods, and paying attention to portion sizes.

This dietary strategy offers a useful tool for those looking to improve their general well-being and make optimal nutritional choices since it places a strong emphasis on the quality of carbohydrates and their effect on the glycemic load.

CHAPTER ONE

Recognition Of Glycemic Load

grasp how different foods affect blood sugar levels requires a grasp of the notion of Glycemic Load (GL).

The concept of Glycemic Load considers the amount and quality of carbs in a given meal item.

Glycemic Load takes into account the actual quantity of carbs taken, whereas Glycemic Index (GI) gauges how rapidly a particular diet elevates blood sugar. This more complex method offers a more thorough comprehension of how diet affects blood sugar.

Glycemic Load: What Is It?

The Glycemic Index of a food is multiplied by the quantity of carbs it contains in a standard serving to determine its Glycemic Load.

This produces a figure that represents the food's total glycemic effect. Low GL foods take longer to digest and absorb, which causes blood sugar levels to rise gradually. Foods with a high GL, on the other hand, quickly raise blood sugar levels.

For those who want to effectively control their blood sugar, Glycemic Load provides more useful advice by taking into account both the type and quantity of carbs.

Glycemic Load And Glycemic Index Different

Making the distinction between Glycemic Index and Glycemic Load is essential for making well-informed dietary decisions.

Glycemic Load gives a more realistic image by taking into consideration the entire amount of carbohydrates in a food, whereas Glycemic Index only considers how quickly a food containing carbohydrates elevates blood sugar. Conversely, if low-GI foods are consumed in big quantities, they can nevertheless have a considerable glycemic impact. High-GI foods may have a more moderate effect on blood sugar if ingested in smaller quantities.

Comprehending this differentiation enables people to make more sophisticated choices about their consumption of carbohydrates.

High Glycemic Load's Effect On Blood Sugar

Consuming foods high in glycemic load may cause blood sugar levels to climb quickly and then plummet. Shortly after eating, this rollercoaster impact may exacerbate sensations of exhaustion, irritation, and hunger.

Insulin resistance, a disorder in which the body's cells lose their insulin sensitivity, may develop over time as a result of frequent exposure to high-glycemic foods. Since persistently high blood sugar levels are linked to an increased risk of type 2 diabetes and other metabolic problems, controlling and stabilizing blood sugar levels is crucial for overall health.

Knowing Glycemic Load offers a more sophisticated method of controlling blood sugar than only using Glycemic Index. Through careful consideration of the type and amount of carbs consumed, people can make well-informed decisions that support stable blood sugar levels and general health.

This knowledge is especially important for anyone trying to avoid or treat diabetes and insulin resistance.

CHAPTER TWO

Low Glycemic Load Diet Benefits

The Low Glycemic Load Diet is a popular dietary strategy that aims to support stable blood sugar levels.

Foods having a low glycemic load—that is, ones that have little effect on blood sugar—are the focus of this diet.

We will examine the advantages of the Low Glycemic Load Diet in this conversation, paying particular attention to how it affects energy levels, mental clarity, weight control, and long-term health.

Control Of Weight

A Low Glycemic Load Diet's beneficial effects on weight management are among its main benefits.

Low-glycemic foods take longer to digest and absorb, which causes blood sugar levels to rise gradually.

This steady rise aids in minimizing overall food consumption and managing hunger. Moreover, low-glycemic foods' prolonged energy supply helps with feelings of fullness, which lowers the risk of overeating and encourages weight loss.

Increased Levels Of Energy

The goal of the low-glycemic load diet is to release energy consistently and sustainably throughout the day. Low-glycemic foods help to maintain a more steady level of energy in contrast to high-glycemic foods, which quickly raise and fall blood sugar levels.

This may be especially helpful for people who feel lethargic or low on energy after eating high-glycemic meals.

Low-glycemic diets provide longer-lasting energy that promotes increased focus, endurance, and productivity.

Improved Intelligence

Improved mental clarity can be facilitated by the Low Glycemic Load Diet, and stable blood sugar levels are strongly associated with improved cognitive performance.

Blood sugar swings can have an impact on memory, focus, and general cognitive function.

People who eat low-glycemic foods may notice improvements in their mood stability and cognitive function. This dietary component is especially important for activities requiring prolonged concentration and mental focus.

Long-Term Advantages For Health

The Low Glycemic Load Diet has long-term health benefits in addition to its immediate effects on energy and weight.

High blood sugar levels regularly are linked to a higher chance of acquiring chronic illnesses including type 2 diabetes and cardiovascular disease. By making low-glycemic foods a priority in their diet, people can lower their chance of developing these conditions and improve their general health.

Long-term improved metabolic health may also be facilitated by this diet's consistent energy and steady blood sugar levels.

The benefits of the Low Glycemic Load Diet go beyond just helping people lose weight quickly.

It offers a comprehensive strategy for keeping blood sugar levels steady.

This dietary approach highlights the significance of selecting foods with a low glycemic load, with benefits ranging from increased energy to better mental clarity and long-term health.

People may see improvements in their physical and mental health by adopting These Ideas Into Their Daily Lives.

How To Make A Low-Glycemic Load Plate

The Low Glycemic Load (GL) diet is a way of eating that emphasizes foods low in glycemic load to help maintain stable blood sugar levels.

Glycemic load is a measure of a food's effect on blood sugar that takes into accounts both the kind and amount of carbs in the food.

Choosing meals that have a low impact on blood sugar levels and arranging them in a balanced way are the first steps in creating a low-glycemic load plate.

Selecting Foods With Low Glycemic Load

The glycemic index (GI) of each food is important to consider when following a Low Glycemic Load diet.

Low-glycemic foods usually take longer to absorb, which causes blood sugar levels to rise gradually.

It is crucial to prioritize complete, unprocessed foods such as fruits, vegetables, lean meats, and whole grains. Because of their reduced glycemic load, these foods offer longer-lasting energy and less chance of blood sugar rises.

Controlled Portioning And Equilibrium Macronutrients

Controlling portion sizes is essential for regulating blood sugar levels.

While selecting foods with a low glycemic load is crucial, eating the right amounts of carbohydrates also helps avoid overdoing it.

Another important component of the Low Glycemic Load diet is balancing macronutrients, such as proteins, fats, and carbohydrates.

Properly combining these nutrients results in a more prolonged release of energy throughout the day and aids in blood sugar regulation.

Preparing Foods High In Nutrients

Making nutrient-dense meals that supply vital vitamins and minerals along with supporting stable blood sugar levels is a fundamental component of the Low Glycemic Load diet.

A wide spectrum of nutrients is ensured by including a mix of vibrant fruits and vegetables, while lean proteins and healthy fats aid with satiety.

Using a variety of herbs and spices to flavor food instead of high-glycemic additives will help create a more healthful and well-balanced diet.

When following a Low Glycemic Load diet, careful planning is needed to create a plate that gives priority to items that have the least negative effect on blood sugar levels.

Foods with a low glycemic load, portion management, and a balance of macronutrients all support stable blood sugar levels and general health.

In addition to helping with blood sugar regulation, preparing nutrient-rich meals guarantees a varied and healthful approach to nutrition.

CHAPTER THREE

Determining Foods With High And Low Glycemic Load

It is essential to comprehend the glycemic load of meals to keep blood sugar levels steady.

The glycemic load provides a more precise assessment of how a certain item affects blood sugar by accounting for both the amount and quality of carbs in a serving.

Foods with a high glycemic load may quickly raise and lower blood sugar levels, which can exacerbate sensations of hunger and exhaustion.

Conversely, foods with a low glycemic load release glucose more gradually, resulting in longer-lasting energy levels.

Foods With A High Glycemic Load To Avoid

High-glycemic foods can cause blood sugar levels to rise quickly, which may result in insulin resistance and other health problems.

Foods that are known to affect blood sugar levels include processed snacks, sugary cereals, and white bread.

By staying away from certain foods with high glycemic loads, people can better control their blood sugar levels and lower their chance of contracting diseases like type 2 diabetes.

Identifying these foods and choosing wisely is crucial for anyone trying to follow a low-glycemic load diet.

Other Low-Glycemic Load Options

Selecting low-glycemic load substitutes is a crucial tactic for encouraging steady blood sugar levels. Legumes, non-starchy veggies, and whole grains are great options that supply vital nutrients without abrupt blood sugar increases.

Lean proteins and good fats can also help to further balance meals and slow down the absorption of carbohydrates.

People can promote their general health and well-being while enjoying a varied and pleasant diet by replacing high glycemic load meals with these options.

Examining Food Labels To Learn About Glycemic Load

Anyone trying to adhere to a low glycemic load diet will find that reading food labels is an invaluable skill.

Comprehending the meaning of glycemic load data on packaging enables shoppers to make knowledgeable decisions at the grocery store.

To determine the glycemic load precisely, look for labels that include information on serving size, fiber content, and total carbohydrates. With this information, people can make more informed meal choices that support their nutritional objectives and improve their general health and blood sugar regulation. More items may list the glycemic load on their labels as consumer understanding of the term rises, facilitating healthy decision-making.

Organizing Meals And Recipes

Effective meal planning is a cornerstone of the Low Glycemic Load diet.

Meal planning during the week guarantees a balanced consumption of lipids, proteins, and carbohydrates while controlling blood sugar levels.

It entails choosing meals with a low Glycemic Load and calculating portion sizes carefully.

Example Meal Plans with Low Glycemic Loads

Making realistic and diverse meal plans is crucial to following the Low Glycemic Load diet. Sample meal plans can be used as a reference, providing people with a structure to follow while creating their weekly menus. To support long-lasting energy and satiety, these diets have a strong emphasis on healthy grains, lean proteins, and an abundance of fruits and vegetables.

Yummy And Healthful Low-Glycemic Load Recipes

Adopting a Low Glycemic Load diet does not imply flavor sacrifice. There are many tasty and nourishing recipes available that are adapted to this type of eating. The culinary alternatives are endless, ranging from supper preparations that feature lean proteins and veggies high in fiber to breakfast ones that incorporate oats and berries.

These dishes appeal to those with discriminating tastes as well as those seeking blood sugar stability.

The Low Glycemic Load diet is a useful tool for people who want to support general health and keep blood sugar levels steady.

By emphasizing thoughtful meal planning and including delicious recipes, this nutritional strategy provides a pleasurable and sustainable means of promoting well-being. People can take proactive measures to achieve and maintain optimal metabolic health by learning the Low Glycemic Load diet principles and applying them to their daily lives.

CHAPTER FOUR

Workout's Impact On Blood Sugar Regulation

Exercise is an important part of a low-glycemic load lifestyle since it is crucial for blood sugar management.

Exercise improves insulin sensitivity, which improves the way cells use glucose. People can modify their fitness regimens to support stable glucose levels by being aware of how exercise affects blood sugar levels.

Exercise And The Control Of Blood Sugar

Exercise regularly directly affects blood sugar management. Engaging in physical exercise causes muscle cells to absorb more glucose, which lowers blood glucose levels.

Resistance training and aerobic exercise both enhance insulin sensitivity, facilitating better blood sugar uptake and storage.

Suggested Exercise Routines

Selecting the appropriate kind of physical activity is crucial for people who want to keep their blood sugar stable.

Walking, running, cycling, and swimming are examples of aerobic exercises that help improve blood sugar regulation and cardiovascular health.

Insulin sensitivity can be further enhanced by adding resistance training, such as weightlifting, which can increase muscle mass.

How To Design A Balanced Exercise Program

Several exercise modalities are combined in a well-rounded fitness regimen to treat specific health issues.

A balanced approach to fitness is achieved by incorporating strength training, flexibility training, and aerobic activity. This variety improves general physical and mental health in addition to improving blood sugar balance.

Regular exercise and the Low Glycemic Load Diet combine to create a potent plan for sustaining stable blood sugar levels.

Not only can people efficiently control their blood sugar levels through dietary choices, meal planning, and participation in a variety of physical activities, but they may also promote long-term health and vitality. Including these ideas in your daily routine will enhance your general health and lower your chance of problems from blood sugar swings.

CHAPTER FIVE

Overcoming Difficulties

Although there are many advantages to the low glycemic load diet, some may find it difficult to incorporate this dietary strategy into their daily routine.

A mix of preparation, resilience, and education is needed to overcome these obstacles.

Practical And Social Difficulties

Keeping up a low-glycemic load diet can be challenging in social and practical contexts.

For instance, a wide range of food alternatives are frequently served at social gatherings, many of which may have a high glycemic index. Proactive planning and efficient communication are necessary to handle these circumstances. Sharing dietary preferences with friends and family and looking into healthier options for group meals may be beneficial.

Advice On Eating Out

For people on a low glycemic load diet, eating out might be challenging because many meals on restaurant menus contain high GI ingredients.

However, it is feasible to follow the guidelines of this nutritional plan and still enjoy dining out if you make wise decisions.

When dining out, choosing lean protein, non-starchy veggies, and healthy grains can help make meals that are low in Glycemic load and well-balanced.

Handling Intense Wants

A common problem for those making the switch to a low-glycemic load diet is cravings for high-glycemic foods.

Effective coping tactics require an understanding of the underlying causes of these urges, such as emotional triggers or ingrained tendencies.

Along with regular meals and snacks, incorporating a range of tasty and filling low-GI foods into the diet will help reduce cravings and encourage long-term adherence to the low-glycemic load lifestyle.

An effective strategy for fostering steady blood sugar levels and general well-being is the low glycemic load diet.

It takes knowledge, preparation, and persistence to overcome obstacles related to social settings, eating out, and cravings. People can take advantage of a low glycemic load diet and effectively manage the challenges of everyday living by implementing these measures.

Keeping An Eye On And Controlling Blood Sugar Levels

Blood sugar regulation is essential for general health, particularly for those with diabetes and other medical disorders. To do this, the Low Glycemic Load (LGL) diet has become an important resource. Consuming foods with a low glycemic load—those that have little effect on blood sugar levels—is the main goal of this dietary strategy. Better blood sugar control can be achieved by comprehending and applying the LGL diet's tenets to daily living.

The Value Of Consistent Monitoring

A vital component of treating diseases like diabetes and following the Low Glycemic Load diet is routine blood sugar monitoring.

Monitoring gives people vital knowledge about how various diets and lifestyle choices impact blood sugar, empowering them to make wise decisions.

Regular tracking makes it easier to spot trends and makes it possible to make timely changes to the diet and other components of the management strategy.

People can prevent problems linked to uncontrolled blood sugar by actively managing swings and preserving stability by closely monitoring their blood sugar levels.

Collaborating With Medical Experts

Working together with medical specialists is essential to successfully controlling blood sugar levels. Healthcare professionals are essential in helping people understand the nuances of the Low Glycemic Load diet and in customizing advice to meet specific needs.

Customized nutrition plan modifications depending on age, weight, exercise level, and any underlying medical concerns are made possible by routine check-ups, consultations, and talks with healthcare professionals.

This collaboration guarantees that people get all the help they need to start and maintain a low-glycemic load diet.

Changing The Diet To Meet Personal Needs

The Low Glycemic Load Diet's adaptability to different needs and levels of flexibility is one of its main advantages.

Each person's body uniquely responds to different foods, and variables like insulin sensitivity and metabolism might range greatly.

 Changing the diet to suit these unique requirements necessitates experimenting with varied meal times, portion sizes, and food selections.

 Having close consultation with a medical professional or qualified dietitian can help you create a Low Glycemic Load diet plan that suits your unique needs and health objectives.

The Low Glycemic Load diet is a useful tool for people who are controlling diabetes or other diseases that require stable blood sugar levels. A good blood sugar management strategy must include regular monitoring, working with healthcare providers, and making customized dietary changes.

By integrating these components into their everyday routines, people can actively work toward reaching and maintaining ideal blood sugar regulation.

CHAPTER SIX

Stories Of Success

Starting a path towards stable blood sugar frequently requires sharing personal success stories that encourage others to make life-improving decisions.

People who follow the Low Glycemic Load Diet spoke about how they overcame obstacles and saw a major increase in their general state of well-being.

These success stories add to the increasing amount of information demonstrating the diet's advantages and serve as a testament to its efficacy in controlling blood sugar levels.

Experiences With The Low Glycemic Load Diet In Real Life

Experiences from the real world provide important context for understanding how the Low Glycemic Load Diet should be used.

This section explores people's daily struggles and how they have dealt with the complexity of dietary choices.

These stories offer an insight into the practical applications of a low glycemic load diet, from meal preparation to social situations.

This post seeks to help and inspire those who are following a similar road by offering these real-life experiences.

Motivating Tales Of Stable Blood Sugar

The path to stable blood sugar is frequently a transformative one, requiring tenacity and dedication.

 The motivational stories of those who have effectively adopted a low-glycemic load diet are examined in this section. These stories, which range from early hardships to significant turning points, demonstrate the tenacity and resolve needed to bring about long-lasting change.

These tales can serve as a source of inspiration for readers, who will also learn important lessons about the revolutionary potential of the low-glycemic load diet.

Conclusion

It appears that the Low Glycemic Load Diet is a viable strategy for preserving steady blood sugar levels.

This article clarifies the effects of diet on people's lives by examining success tales, actual experiences, and motivational journeys.

With increased awareness of the benefits of stable blood sugar for general health, the Low Glycemic Load Diet presents a workable and realistic alternative that gives hope and inspiration to anyone looking for a long-term way to better health.

One useful strategy for encouraging steady blood sugar levels is the Low

Glycemic Load Diet. Its focus on choosing foods with a reduced glycemic load helps to promote satiety, maintain energy levels throughout the day, and improve overall glycemic control.

Although it could necessitate careful meal preparation and a certain level of nutritional mindfulness, the long-term advantages make it a good choice for people who want to control their blood sugar and improve their general health.

Comprehending the fundamentals of the Low Glycemic Load Diet is imperative for its effective execution.

The importance of glycemic load and index, the choice of low-glycemic foods, careful meal preparation, and the possible effects on blood sugar regulation and weight control are among the main lessons to be learned. People who use these guidelines can make well-informed decisions that support the objectives of the Low Glycemic Load Diet.

Motivation For Extended-Term Compliance

Commitment is necessary for any dietary adjustment, and the Low Glycemic Load Diet is no different.

It is possible to promote long-term adherence to this eating pattern by progressively implementing its principles into daily life, experimenting with different recipes and food combinations, and getting advice from nutritionists or medical professionals.

Acknowledging the benefits for general health and well-being provides an incentive for continued adherence, which is why the Low Glycemic Load Diet is a useful strategy for people who want to stabilize their blood sugar and improve their quality of life.